THE 21ST CENTURY VIRGINS: CLOSED LEGS

THERESA FULLER

ABSTRACT:

This book is aimed especially at virgin ladies who are not aware of the occurrence in their systems, especially in the vagina area. The book will also help you get prepare for the things that would happen in real life.

Table of Contents

Numerous youngsters are extremely hopeful about marriage; at any rate, that is the impression I get when I collaborate with them. At a young assembling at some point back, a young fellow recounted to me this story and requested exhortation. His companion and his life partner had concurred that there will be no early sex, chiefly on the demand of the woman.

The young fellow hesitantly concurred and anticipated ravishing his better half in the wake of the wedding, however unfortunately he experienced no barrier on their most memorable excursion. He was irate and disheartened. He then asked me, how should his companion respond.

It was my chance to fire him. "Did the woman tell your spouse during courtship that she was a virgin?" He addressed no. So the companion just expected. "What or who is your partner getting married to, the virginity or the lady?"

"The woman," he replied. "So the issue lies with what? This companion who is fixated on virginity, is he a virgin?" The reaction was "no." A lot of the time we seek shadows instead of substance.

Then, at that point, I recollected a story another companion let me know some time prior and I began pondering, who is a virgin? My companion said in a specific nation (name kept because I couldn't freely confirm his story), it is wrongdoing or untouchable for an inexperienced lady to misplace her "virginity" before marriage.

So what the young ladies do is participate in the butt-centric entrance (Also known as butt-centric sex) and the men likewise grab their bosoms, bums and different pieces of their bodies during pre-intimate relationships. Be that as it may, their hymen (the film to some degree or covering the launch of the vagina) is still there for their future spouses to "gladly" break after marriage. My inquiry is: are these young ladies still virgins?

Additionally in certain connections where life partners and life partners consent to no sex before marriage, they participate in all types of physically private demonstrations, aside from real vaginal entrance with the penis; would they say they are still virgins? Some lesbians are effectively associated with same-sex connections, yet have never been entered, so their hymen may be flawless, would they say they are virgins?

Presently it gets somewhat confounded. A way of thinking contends that assault casualties, who were virgins before the assault, are still virgins, even though they have been entered and the hymen, broken. They contend that as long as they didn't agree to the demonstration, they are virgins since assent is essential for losing your virginity.

We know beyond a shadow of a doubt that sports ladies and others engaged with a few proactive tasks can unintentionally break their hymen. The ramifications are that there is no proof to demonstrate their virginity, however, could those of them who at any point have never engaged in sexual relations be delegated virgins?

Who is a virgin? The basic word reference meaning of a virgin is "an individual who has never had sex." So what is sex? Wikipedia says sex "is chiefly the inclusion and pushing of a male's penis, generally when erect, into a female's vagina... "

 This definition is old, customary and doesn't address arising patterns.

Mankind has "moved" on. Same-sex connections and relationships have been sanctioned in numerous nations, a reality Wikipedia recognizes. In this way, sex presently incorporates "oral sex," "butt-centric sex" and "fingering" among numerous other recent fads.

So who is a virgin? The meaning of a virgin has turned into a question of individual translations to many, however, I will connect virginity with one who is unadulterated, modest, unsullied, unpolluted and pure. You make your derivations.

Numerous young fellows need to wed virgins, yet can't track down them. Water all over the place, yet none to drink. Who are the poisons? For what reason are the virgins scant? We as a whole know. Assuming wedded people let single men and old maids be and unhitched males and old maids keep their hands off each other, there will be a torrential slide of virgins. We are thumping our heads over a circumstance we contributed to making?

To young fellows searching for "virgins" to wed, this is my take. It is your life and you reserve an option to live it how you like inside legitimate cut-off points, obviously, yet I disapprove of individuals who come to value with foul hands. Additionally, what precisely do you need from marriage? You should have clearness of direction, with the goal that you don't zero in on the vaporous to the impairment of repeating issues in marriage.

Virginity is an ideal and it is great for otherworldly reasons and the vibe great component, however, offenders ought to be pardoned.

God's elegance, if not, I won't be here flapping my gums, sorry pen.

I have a place with bunches who urge youngsters to carry on with virtuous lives, yet we don't censure other people who have committed errors, since "there is no judgment unto the people who are in Christ Jesus.

Allow me to finish up with a similarity. Earlier expressions of remorse for contrasting God's made and synthetic articles, however, I see a connection between virgins/non-virgins and fresh-out-of-the-box new vehicles/genuinely utilized vehicles. Everyone cherishes a fresh box new vehicle. We love the newness, the pride of being the individual who detached the "elastic," however might everyone at any point bear the cost of a fresh box new vehicle?

Once more on the off chance that you are offered a shiny new Kia Picanto and a Lexus Jeep that has done just 5000 miles, which one will you pick? Likewise, between a pristine Honda Accord and a Rolls Royce with a 10,000 mileage, which offers unrivalled execution?

Which is better, wedding a virgin you will live fiercely with until the end of your life or a companion who is a perfect partner, even though she had an earlier relationship? Virginity is great, authentic and sacred, however, marriage is significantly more than virginity. Marriage as of now has trailer-heaps of issues. Figure out earlier issues during romance and leave them there; don't bring them into marriage.

CHAPTER 1

Myths

Virginity is many times introduced in straightforward, highly contrasting terms: have you engaged in sexual relations, or have you not?

Yet, virginity is a muddled idea that has a long way from one definition. That is because virginity is not a clinical idea. What you consider virginity typically relies upon your social foundation and strict childhood. This multitude of thoughts regarding virginity (joined with an absence of sex training overall) intends that there is a ton of falsehood out there about what virginity is, and who is or alternately is not a virgin. The following are 7 normal fantasies about virginity, and what you want to be aware of all things considered.

1. Virginity is either/or.

Individuals frequently discuss virginity like it has a firm definition: You're either a virgin or you're not. However, virginity is a thought, and it implies various things to various individuals. For instance, some think that individuals are virgins until they've had a penis in vagina (PIV) sex, while others contend that oral sex (going down on, eating out, sensual caress), manual sex (fingering, hand work), or butt-centric sex "count." Others imagine that you're presently not a virgin after you've had your most memorable climax. Various individuals unexpectedly consider virginity. Its definition isn't firmly established. That implies that you can imagine virginity how you need to think about it (if you need to think about it by any means)!

Yet, in case it wasn't already obvious, clinical suppliers think these sex acts to be the genuine article. Since you don't believe a demonstration to be "genuine" sex, doesn't mean you can't get a physically communicated contamination (STI) from it. So when your primary care physician inquires as to whether you're physically dynamic, ensure you say "OK" on the off chance that you're having any sort of sex. Your supplier couldn't care less about the obscure thought of virginity — they care about your wellbeing and engaging you to deal with yourself.

2. Any sort of infiltration (counting a tampon) counts.
Do you believe that embedding a tampon considers having intercourse? No? Then you can't lose your virginity by utilizing a tampon.

3. Specialists can figure out whether you're a virgin.
Clinical suppliers can't tell whether you've had intercourse, whether you have a penis or a vagina. Many individuals believe that specialists can determine if somebody with a vagina has engaged in sexual relations by taking a gander at their hymen, and checking whether it's been torn. However, this is misleading. The hymen is a slim piece of skin tissue that somewhat covers the vaginal opening, frequently (however not generally) in a half-moon shape. During adolescence, hymens become more flexible. Hymens can tear for a wide range of reasons, including doing the parts, embedding a tampon or, indeed, having PIV sex. It is undeniably challenging, and frequently unimaginable, to sort out whether or not a hymen has been torn before. Furthermore, frequently, they won't ever tear! All things considered, the hymen extends — similar to a flexible hair band.

The facts confirm that hymen incidentally (however once in a long while) cover the entire vaginal opening. This is called a flawless hymen, and it tends to be fixed with a minor medical procedure. It is likewise interesting. Consider it: if hymens covered the entire vaginal opening, how might period blood escape?

4. Accomplices can tell.

Sexual accomplices can't figure out if you've had intercourse previously. Many individuals with a vagina don't drain whenever they first have PIV sex (see underneath), and vaginas don't "get free" from sex. Once more, the main way your accomplice will be aware if you're a virgin is on the off chance that you tell them. On the off chance that you're stressed over your accomplice knowing you're a virgin (or knowing you're not a virgin), wonder why. Could it be said that you are apprehensive about their response? Could it be said that they are tolerating and getting it? Have you discussed sex previously? We've expressed it previously and we'll say it once more: correspondence is a vital piece of sex. While your sexual history is your business and your business alone, having an anxious outlook on your accomplice's response to it could be an indication that sex with this individual (or right now in your life) isn't the most ideal choice.

5. Outsiders can tell.

Is it safe to say that you are detecting an example here? Others can't determine whether you are a virgin. Engaging in sexual relations doesn't meaningfully impact how you walk. Except if you explicitly tell them, they can. not. know.

6. Virgins (who have a vagina) will drain their most memorable time.

While the facts confirm that certain individuals with vaginas drain during PIV sex, it is certainly not guaranteed. As we referenced previously, a great many people's hymen doesn't tear during sex, they stretch. Yet, a ton of young ladies have been instructed that their "first time" will be excruciating and include blood. This naturally makes many individuals anxious, which prompts tenser muscles during sex and an absence of grease. This can cause some vaginal draining and torment. Yet, there are a lot of ways of keeping away from this: go sluggish, include loads of foreplay, snatch some lube, and impart.

7. After you've "lost" your virginity, sex is no biggie. American culture's fixation on virginity infers a large number that first-time, sex is not a problem. In any case, that is simply false. We've discussed how sex is strong, and that turns out as expected every time you have intercourse. Since somebody has given assent once doesn't imply that they're alright engaging in sexual relations once more. Having intercourse with one individual doesn't imply that they're alright having intercourse with any other person.

Individuals decide to have intercourse for a wide range of reasons, and they decide to quit having intercourse for a wide range of reasons as well. Sex isn't a train that you get on and can't get off. YOU get to decide whether you have a sexual coexistence and what it resembles — whether you've had intercourse previously.

CHAPTER 2

Considerations

Suppose you've been dating somebody for some time and you're examining the possibility of having intercourse interestingly together. You're normally feeling pretty eager to take things to a higher level, and you two are discussing how it will go down. Everything looks OK!

In any case, that is when things veer off in a strange direction. She stops and afterwards raises an uncommon muddling point of interest: she's never really done this. Actually no, not simply with you: she's never had intercourse with anybody, period. That is correct — she's a virgin.

How would you continue? What are the guidelines here? How would you cause her to feel as good as could be expected, and ensure her most memorable experience works out positively?

1. Society Has a Ton of Unusual Thoughts Regarding Virginity

The possibility of "virginity" is treated in a wide range of courses in the public eye and through the traditional press, from a humiliation to be disposed of no matter what to a definitive condition of immaculateness and honesty.

By and large, these differentiating originations of virginity partition down orientation lines: men who are virgins are bound to be considered meriting compassion toward their "humiliating" quandary, while female virgins are bound to be viewed as a definitive ideal in immaculateness and guiltlessness. Accepting that the virgin you're considering laying down with is female, it merits considering the entire host of cultural strains she is probably looking at about the idea of her virginity, and what losing it implies.

Likewise worth calculating the thought it's a definitive objective for men to "take" a lady's virginity. It's a dreadful perspective, and it would be smart for you to promise her that that is not your outlook.

2. This May Be a Truly Significant Second for Her (Or Perhaps It Isn't)

Individuals have shifting levels of wistfulness about losing their virginity. For certain individuals - as referenced above, typically guys - virginity is something to be disposed of rapidly and without an excess of show. For other people - normally females, yet not consistently - virginity is a valuable state to be lost just when you've found somebody you genuinely love. For others still, it isn't so much that enormous an arrangement one way or another: it's a nonpartisan occasion; a typical and predictable piece of growing up.

The key thing is for you to decide how your accomplice feels, and continue as needs be from that point. On the off chance that this is a monstrous, gigantic arrangement for her, you will have to discuss it exhaustively and invest some energy in establishing the groundwork for the occasion. Assuming it's not a problem for her, you'll in any case be delicate and kind, yet there might be less close-to-home prep work included. Tailor your way to deal with the disposition of your accomplice, however, decide in favour of regarding it as a huge occasion for her.

3. On the off chance that There Is a Major Age Hole Between You, Think about Not Getting it done

There are loads of reasons that ladies might turn out to be in their 20s or past despite everything in virginal states, at the same time, by and large, virginity will in general connect with a more youthful age.

On the off chance that you are mulling over laying down with a lot more youthful virgin than you (in her teenagers, say, while you are very much into your 20s or more seasoned), it merits rethinking the power elements at play in your circumstance. In some cases little kids like laying down with more seasoned men and may feel as though it causes them to appear to be more fully grown and created than their friends, yet it's typical for them to lament having intercourse with more established men later down the line.

Essentially, this one boils down to everyday courtesy and presumably does without saying for most Ask Men peruses: Don't be a jerk and don't exploit somebody a lot more youthful than you. Ensure the power elements in your relationship are equivalent, and that everybody is completely glad to continue.

4. Discuss Your Assumptions

Are you two in a relationship, or is this something relaxed for you (or her)? Will your relationship go on after you two have intercourse, and to what limit? These are significant issues to manage quite a bit early - you want to ensure everybody is in total agreement and nobody is being set up for hurt thereafter.

You can't forestall one of you getting injured sentiments or lamenting what occurred, however, you can decrease the possibilities with clear, genuine correspondence front and centre.

5. Play it safe to Forestall Undesirable Pregnancy and STIs

Laying down with a virgin doesn't mean you can disregard the standard safety measures you want to take to forestall undesirable pregnancies and the spread of STIs. There are still dangers to consider regardless of who you are laying down with, so ensure you are utilizing assurance (for example condoms) and sufficient contraception, except if you maintain that her most memorable time should be substantially more sensational than it should be.

6. You Should Accept Things Gradually and Tenderly

No matter what your accomplice's demeanour towards losing her virginity, as far as the actual demonstration itself, it will pay to gradually take things.

Sex is something she hasn't encountered previously and she will be genuinely unused to it, which could mean a touch of blood on your sheets and possibly some torment for her. Follow your accomplice: dial back or stop when she tells you to, and pay attention to what she shares with you as far as how she's inclined.

Give additional consideration to non-verbal signals, as well: if she looks like she's awkward, pause and check-in, and check whether there's anything she'd like you to do any other way. This moment isn't the opportunity to explore different avenues regarding wild positions and supported sex long-distance races, and your fundamental spotlight ought to be on guaranteeing your accomplice's solace.

It's memorable essential that the actual sex may not be astounding: it's her most memorable time and considering all the social and cultural around virginity, it's profoundly conceivable that the actual occasion will be a disappointment.

Try not to stress a lot over that side of things: Sex gets better with training, so for her most memorable time, centre around ensuring she's agreeable and blissful.

7. Show up for Her A short time later

No matter what your relationship status is, you ought to be thoughtful and polite to your accomplice in the fallout of her most memorable sexual experience. Nestle, express kind things and stick around. Ensure they return home without a scratch. Ensure she's inclined alright, and monitor how she's inclined tomorrow, as well. Be a helpful individual and a sounding board, and be open about any feelings of dread or concerns you have, as well - she ought to put forth a comparable attempt to ensure that you are feeling emphatically about the experience too.

8. Ensure That You're Having a good sense of security, Blissful and Agreeable, As well

The spotlight here will fundamentally be on your accomplice, as she is the person who is losing her virginity, however, that doesn't mean you drop good and are gone totally. Since you've done this previously, it doesn't mean you don't have to think about your sentiments.

Are things moving quicker than you'd like them to? Is it true or not that you are being forced out of utilizing insurance, or compelled into a relationship you've clarified you don't need? That is not OK, and you're qualified to draw clear limits and support yourself. Once more, correspondence is significant here: ensure you are being completely clear about your assumptions, needs and needs a long time before you two carry out the thing.

The overall objective here is to ensure that both of you have a protected and charming time. Your accomplice will presumably require more planning than you will, and it's your job to show up for her to examine any issues that emerge. She plays a corresponding part to pay attention to your interests, as well as addressing them overall quite well.

So that's it. Laying down with a virgin can be the pretty plague, because of the serious level of strain we put on the idea in any case. However, it needn't bother to be a nervousness-instigating experience. You can ensure it's essentially as sure as workable for you two by acting with deference and nobility, and by keeping the channels of correspondence transparent. Best of luck!

Losing your virginity can appear to be startling, and the scope of fantasies encompassing it doesn't help. While certain ladies might encounter torment during their most memorable involvement in penetrative sex, you mustn't have a terrible time. Conversing with your accomplice and understanding how sex functions can assist you with unwinding in advance. By setting the right state of mind and utilizing the right instruments, you can make your most memorable time a positive and, surprisingly, charming experience.

1.Ensure you are prepared to have intercourse.
Having an anxious outlook on your most memorable time is typical. If you feel tense when you contemplate sex or when you and your accomplice are wasting time, it very well may be an indication that you ought to pause. On the off chance that you have intercourse when it doesn't feel right, you might appreciate sex less and become tense during the demonstration.

Many individuals grow up being shown sex is despicable, ought to be saved for marriage, and is just to be capable between a man and a lady. Assuming that sex causes you to feel regretful or pushed, perhaps you ought to stand by. Have a go at conversing with somebody about your sentiments.

Having high expectations about your body is typical. Yet, on the off chance that you are terrified or can't be exposed given what you look like, it very well may be an indication that you're not exactly prepared to accompany an accomplice.

Try not to feel embarrassed about your sexual inclinations. No one but you can conclude who you're drawn to and what kind of sex you need. Everyone has cut-off points and inclinations, so don't feel regretful about them.

2. Speak with your accomplice.

 Chatting with your accomplice can lay out trust while assisting you with having a more uplifting perspective on having intercourse. A decent accomplice ought to be circumspect of your sentiments and able to help you through the cycle. Assuming that your potential accomplice pressures you to an extreme or causes you to feel awkward, revaluate engaging in sexual relations with them.

On the off chance that pregnancy is plausible, discuss conception prevention and insurance before you engage in sexual relations. You could affirm, "I'm on prevention, yet I would like for you to in any circumstance employ a condom."

Tell them what your apprehensions and assumptions are and the way that you're feeling. You could say, "I'm super apprehensive about it harming the initial time."

Let your accomplice know if there's something you have any desire to attempt or something you don't have any desire to do. For example, you can watch them, "I like oral sex, nonetheless I'm not interested in butt-centric."

Assuming that you're apprehensive or restless, let them know. Assuming that they excuse your sentiments, it could be an indication that they don't seriously view your interests.

3. Find a believed grown-up you can converse with.

 You could feel off-kilter examining sex with a grown-up, however, you ought to essentially distinguish somebody you can contact for help. This could be a parent, a specialist, a nurturer, a school instructor, or more established kin. They can offer you guidance, answer your inquiries, and give admittance to security. Regardless of whether you wind up conversing with them in advance, you might need to have somebody you could contact in the event of a crisis.

On the off chance that you feel constrained to have intercourse, converse with a confided-in grown-up for help. Recall that you never must have sex except if you have any desire to. Nobody ought to pressure you into doing something you would rather not.

Instructing Yourself About Your Body

1.Find out about how sex functions. Understanding your living structures can assist you with feeling more sure, particularly if your accomplice is likewise a virgin. Realizing what goes where, what's typical, and what's in store can assist with facilitating your tension. A few spots you can look at incorporate Arranged Being a parent, Sex, And so on and Carleen.

Masturbation can assist you with understanding what you appreciate about sex. Before engaging in sexual relations with an accomplice, take a stab at trying different things with yourself.

2. Find your hymen.

Despite prevalent thinking, the hymen layer doesn't as a rule cover the vaginal opening except if a condition exists, for example, a micro perforated or septate hymen. As opposed to it being a "mark of newness" in the same way as others say, it is rather the muscle and skin encompassing the opening, likened to the skin and muscle of the butthole. It doesn't "break", yet it very well may be harmed by anything from tampons, doing the parts, or while having intercourse or embedding bigger articles in, which causes the aggravation most virgins feel.

If the hymen is harmed or torn, it will no doubt drain. This should be visible while and after sex. How much blood ought not to be close to as much blood as though you were on your period?

Tearing/"breaking" your hymen ought not to be extremely agonizing. Torment during sex is generally brought about by contact. This can occur if you are not greased up or sufficiently stimulated.

3.Recognize the point of your vagina.
 If you can assist your join forces with slipping into you at the right point, you'll keep away from some possibly excruciating mishandling. Most vaginas are calculated with a forward slant toward the midsection. If you were standing, your vagina would be at a 45-degree point to the floor.
If you use tampons, observe how you approach embedding a tampon. Attempt to reproduce that equivalent point when you start penetrative sex.
On the off chance that you don't utilize tampons, embed a finger whenever you're in the shower. Point toward your lower back; if that feels awkward, shift forward marginally until you find an agreeable point.

experience climax from entrance alone. All things considered, clitoral excitement as a rule makes them climax. Oral sex or clitoral excitement before entrance can loosen up the muscles. Attempt to find your clitoris before you have intercourse. You can do this by jerking off or by looking with a mirror and a spotlight. This can assist you with directing your accomplice to it during sex, particularly if your accomplice is likewise a virgin. Climaxing before infiltration may assist with diminishing torment during sex. Attempt to take part in oral sex during foreplay and before the entrance. Your accomplice can likewise invigorate your clitoris with their fingers or a sex toy.

<u>**Having a ball During Sex**</u>

1.Pick a tranquil area.
If you're continually stressed over getting found out, you probably won't have a good time. Make it more straightforward for yourself and your accomplice by picking an overall setting where you will not be upset.
Search for security, an agreeable surface to rest on, and when you're not stressed over being on a timetable.
Ponder whether you're happier with engaging in sexual relations at your place or theirs.
Assuming you're in a residence or on the other hand assuming that you share a room, you could request that your flatmate give you some time alone that evening.

2.Set a loosening up mind-set.
 Relax by making the climate tranquil. Tidy up any diverting mess, shut off your telephone, and eliminate anything more that could cause you to feel apprehensive or hold you back from zeroing in on your accomplice.
Faint lighting, delicate music, and a warm room temperature can assist with causing you to have a good sense of reassurance and agreement.
Consider setting aside some margin to prepare yourself ahead of time so you feel loose and sure.

have straightforwardly consented to engage in sexual relations. If you don't know how your accomplice is feeling, ask before going ahead. Since your accomplice doesn't say "no," it doesn't mean you have asserted. They ought to answer with a sure, outright "yes."

If your accomplice doesn't need sex, don't pressure them. On the off chance that you don't need sex, they ought to ease off when you say no.

Assent additionally implies that you shouldn't do anything that your accomplice isn't energetic about.

4.

Use insurance. Insurance safeguards against both pregnancy and additionally physically communicated diseases (STIs). Utilizing security might assist you with unwinding on the off chance that you are anxious about getting pregnant or having an illness. Different types of conception prevention don't safeguard against STIs, so assurance provides you with an additional layer of insurance. Assuming your accomplice will not utilize assurance, you might need to revaluate engaging in sexual relations with them.

Condoms aren't the main sort of security! Assuming your accomplice will perform oral sex on you, tight clamp versa, you ought to utilize dental dams and safeguard against sexually transmitted diseases.

There are both male/outer and female/inner condoms accessible.

Assuming you want to purchase condoms, the main thing about condoms is that they fit. Accomplices ought to purchase perhaps one or two sorts of condoms. Give them a shot and see what fits best. On the off chance that your accomplice has a plastic sensitivity, nitrile condoms are an extraordinary other option.

On the off chance that pregnancy is plausible, condoms ought to be worn previously, during, and after entrance. This will expand your security against STIs and pregnancy.

5.
Apply grease.
Grease will facilitate a ton of aggravation by lessening erosion.
It can likewise assist with keeping condoms from breaking
during sex. Apply oil to your accomplice's penis over the
condom or sex toy before they enter you.
If you're utilizing plastic condoms, don't utilize an oil-based oil.
These can debilitate the plastic and prompt the condom to tear
or break. All things considered, utilize a silicone-or water-based
lube. Utilizing any sort of lube with a nitrile or polyurethane
condom is protected.

6
Take as much time as necessary.
Attempt to partake in the second as opposed to hurrying to the
end goal. Invest energy in sorting out what you and your
accomplice both appreciate. Begin with kissing, move to make
out, and adhere to anything pace feels generally good for both
of you.
Foreplay can assist you with unwinding while at the same time
expanding excitement. It can likewise expand your normal
grease, making it simpler for your accomplice to effortlessly
enter you.
Recollect that you can quit engaging in sexual relations
anytime. Assent is dynamic and continuous. You reserve the
privilege to stop or pull out assent anytime you need.

7
Impart your requirements.
 Don't hesitate for even a moment to request what you want at
the time. In the case something feels much better, let your
accomplice know. Assuming that something is causing you

agony or distress, tell them. They ought to take the necessary steps to cause you to feel delighted rather than torment.

Assuming you're feeling torment, have a go at dialling back, moving all the more tenderly, or utilizing more grease. For instance, assuming that you feel torment, you could say, "Would you care if we delayed? This is harming me at present." You can inquire as to whether the one you're utilizing is awkward. For instance, assuming you are on top of your accomplice, you can all the more likely control the speed and point of entrance.

8
Do some aftercare.
 If you have torment or dying, manage it before it turns out to be excessively tyrannical. Take an over-the-counter pain killer, tidy up any blood, and wear a light cushion for a couple of hours. If you experience outrageous torment, you want to converse with a believed grown-up or see a medical services supplier.

Question
For what reason do I begin to shake each time my sweetheart and I intend to engage in sexual relations?

You may not exactly be prepared to engage in sexual relations yet, or you might be terrified. Contemplate assuming you are prepared to engage in sexual relations. Is it true or not that you are adequately adult? Is it true or not that you are feeling forced to have intercourse? Do you truly think often about your accomplice and does he treat you well and truly care about you? On the off chance that you don't think you are prepared at this point, converse with your accomplice and request that he hold on until you are. If you are prepared and have a mindful accomplice, discuss why you might be frightened. On the off chance that you are stressed over pregnancy or sicknesses, ensure you use condoms and go on to conception prevention first. On the off chance that you are frightened of agony, read the article for tips.

Question
How would you forestall pregnancy?

On the off chance that you will have intercourse, the most effective way to forestall pregnancy is to begin taking the pill or Depo shot a little while before you have intercourse, AND utilize a condom too like clockwork. Assuming that you take the pill, you need to ensure you take it when you should every day and not miss pills. Furthermore, assuming you do the Depo shot, you need to get it when it's expected, about like clockwork.

Tips
If you experience horrifying torment or weighty dying, consider a specialist to be as soon as could be expected.
On the off chance that you feel like this evening isn't "the evening," don't be embarrassed to stand by. A mindful accomplice will esteem how you feel above anything more. Assuming you adjust your perspective, it is alright to say as much!

You could get the inclination to go to the latrine during sex. This is typical. Peeing before sex can ease this sensation. Assuming you experience this with a vacant bladder, you might be somebody who can encounter female discharge.

Admonitions
Try not to surrender to tension from your accomplice. It's your choice, not any other individual's.
Drink or remove no sort of medication from dread of torment. It could exacerbate it.

Assuming that your accomplice has had numerous accomplices, you ought to request that they get tried for STIs. STIs are spread through vaginal, butt-centric, and oral sex.

 Individuals can convey and pass on STIs without showing side effects. You can diminish your possibilities of getting a sexually transmitted disease by utilizing condoms, dental dams, and other hindrance techniques.

If you take contraception pills and are taking different drugs, for example, antimicrobials, this can at times change the impacts of the pill. Continuously counsel your primary care physician before beginning any drugs to check whether there will be any regrettable connections with your conception prevention.
It is feasible to get pregnant whenever you first engage in sexual relations. Condoms are profoundly viable when utilized accurately, however on the off chance that conceivable, you ought to utilize one more type of conception prevention alongside a condom

1
What occurs after you lose your virginity?

Losing virginity is an enormous issue, particularly in a nation like our own. After your most memorable sex, you might have a lot of worries about your body. Other than the hymen, which doesn't wind up 'breaking' as a rule, there are numerous different changes that a lady's body goes through post their most memorable sexual experience. Here are some of them:

2
Vaginal changes

VAGINAL CHANGES: The flexibility of your vagina changes after you begin having intercourse. Since the vagina is as yet becoming acclimated to this new movement you have acquainted with your body, it requires investment for the vagina to become used to infiltration. In any case, this gets better with time. Indeed, even the way that your vagina greases up itself will change throughout some period.

3
Clitoris and uterus know when to contract and grow

CLITORIS AND UTERUS KNOW WHEN TO Agreement AND Grow: When in an exciting position, your clitoris will puff up and the uterus will rise a little. After some time, your body will become used to sex and each time you stir, your generally dormant clitoris and uterus will go through these changes and return to typical post the demonstration.

4
Boobs become firmer

Boobs BECOME FIRMER: During and after sex, the tissues in your bosom puff up and the veins expand prompting firmer bosoms. Yet, this returns to typical post-sex and is just a transient state.

5
You experience vasocongestion...

Vasocongestion is the expansion of substantial tissues which are brought about by an expanded vascular blood stream which prompts the bosom, areolas, labia and clitoris to become extended. During this sexual excitement, very much oxygenated blood is provided to your private parts and bosoms. Thus, the external lips, inward lips and clitoris might start to grow and your pulse and circulatory strain may likewise increment quickly.

6
Your skin might begin gleaming

Indeed, you read that right. This is one of the covered-up yet genuinely astonishing advantages of losing your virginity. At the point when you have intercourse for the absolute first time, it might straightforwardly affect the gleam all over - particularly assuming the demonstration got done with a climax. The rationale is basic, when you engage in sexual relations, it further develops your blood dissemination, which helps in siphoning oxygen to your skin, giving it that great, energetic sparkle. Additionally, when you engage in sexual relations, your cerebrum discharges cheerful chemicals like Serotonin and Oxycontin, which help in chopping down the feelings of anxiety and cause you to feel loose. The outcome? You get more clear-looking skin with a lit-from-inside shine.

7
Areolas become more touchy than overall

Areolas BECOME MORE Touchy Overall: When you begin enjoying sex, your body goes through various new encounters. The blood course around your areolas increments and the strong pressure increments make them more delicate than expected.

8
Cheerful hormones

Cheerful hormones: Blissful chemicals are the justification for that gleaming skin. Accordingly, the vibe great chemical of your body, serotonin, gets emitted. Other than this, when you climax, it delivers one more chemical known as oxytocin, which causes you to feel cheerful and loose.

9
Postpone in periods

Postpone IN PERIODS: Since your chemicals get dynamic, there are chances your period might get deferred. Fret not, this isn't a pregnancy caution but instead your body's approach to letting you know that it's going through changes.

10
Intense subject matters

Intense subject matters: Post losing your virginity, you might have close-to-home explosions, both blissful and miserable. This is because of the hormonal changes and can cause you to feel the limits of both of the feelings.

11
Does the initial time hurt?

Keep in mind, that everybody's most memorable time is an alternate encounter, yet it means quite a bit to utilize security to forestall pregnancy and sexually transmitted diseases. At the point when you engage in sexual relations interestingly, it might damage or feel awkward, because of the absence of oil, inferable from the grating. If sex keeps on being agonizing for you, you can attempt various points or positions to lessen the distress and request that your accomplice goes sluggish about the regard. Continuously look for specialist guidance on the off chance that sex keeps on leftover difficult.

12
Practice safe sex

Losing one's virginity holds extraordinary importance for some. In any case, you actually should don't lose your sanity in that energy. Ensure you practice safe sex by utilizing a condom, dental dams, or potentially plastic or nitrile gloves.

Physically sent illnesses (sexually transmitted diseases) may prompt low quality of life, making you more inclined to conceptive issues from here on out.

1

Does eating garlic, or onions deteriorate the vaginal smell?

Once in a while, the smell of our vaginas goes bad and they become things we don't want to smell by any means. However there is a sure smell to it and the vaginal release, that isn't disagreeable. Be that as it may, when it starts to smell odd, it can lead you to worry. All in all, for what motive does this happen?

2

Reasons for change in the smell of vagina

Reasons for CHANGE IN THE SMELL OF VAGINA: Many reasons can prompt an adjustment of the smell of your vagina, including sweat, unfortunate cleanliness, certain ailments, for example, bacterial vaginosis and trichomoniasis, and even food!

3

Food and vaginal smell

FOOD AND VAGINAL SMELL: What you eat can affect how your vagina smells. If you eat solid-smelling food varieties, for example, onions and garlic, it can prompt an impactful smelling vagina. Going against the norm, assuming you eat sweet food varieties like pineapple, your vagina is probably going to smell better.

4
For what reason does this occur?
For what reason DOES THIS Occur? Your vagina fosters an unmistakable smell when there is a bacterial irregularity. Whatever upsets the ordinary acidic equilibrium of your vagina can prompt the improvement of a smell. Frequently, it very well may be because of regular factors like sex or food sources however it can likewise be disturbed because of variables like bacterial contaminations.

5
How long will the smell last?
HOW LONG WILL THE SMELL LAST? In typical cases, the smell ought to fully recover in 48 hours or less. To make the interaction last more limited, you can have heaps of water with the goal that your body flushes out the smell. Be that as it may, on the off chance that the smell continues past 72 hours, you should look for a specialist as it very well may be a sign of a more serious disease.

CHAPTER 5

No announcement

Jessica, a 23-year-old who lives in Mississippi, was dating a person as of late when the subject of sexual history came up. "He was making me understand that he was a virgin and that he intended to hold on until he's tied," she said. "And afterwards he was like, would you say you are a virgin, as well?"

Jessica said she promptly felt anxious. She'd had intercourse previously, but since of her strict convictions, had since been avoiding sex. "It was nerve-wracking," she said. "It was difficult, on the stand that there was no breeze for me. At times it seems like it's acceptable for folks to do whatever, yet if a young lady says, no I'm not a virgin, we're taken a gander at with more disgrace."

That incorporated disgrace is something that a ton of young ladies tragically experience — paying little heed to the strict foundation. What's more, Jessica's right that people are dealt with distinctively about sexual history. If it's not very noticeable in mainstream society, endless examinations report a sexual twofold norm. Hetero men are by and large compensated for having a bigger number of sexual accomplices, while ladies are vilified for the same thing.

So it seems OK that ladies are concerned, as was Jessica, about letting another sexual accomplice know whether they've had intercourse previously. It's difficult to know precisely the number of ladies that vibe restless about this, yet the initial not many autofill results on both Google and Yippee! Answers demonstrate that worry about uncovering sexual history is normal.

What's more, obviously it is, because joined with the unavoidable twofold standard that says folks will possibly like you assuming that you're an unadulterated, virginal heavenly messenger who's never had intercourse before is the legend that whether you drain after sex will part with your sexual history.

To facilitate any of those worries: It's to a great extent false that each lady drains after first-time sex. That centre school gossip comes from a misconception of the hymen, or a flimsy piece of tissue situated about centimetres inside the vaginal opening. Assuming that you've heard the expression "cherry popped" (an expression that totally should be killed and never revived, coincidentally), it's a shoptalk term for the hymen "breaking" after first-time penetrative sex. However, as this site has made sense of previously, the hymen never as a matter of fact "breaks." It extends, and for about a portion, everything being equal, this occurs during another, non-sexual action (like bouncing on a trampoline or riding a bicycle), in many cases in youth.

Indeed, a few ladies experience light to direct draining in the wake of having intercourse interestingly. Yet, draining can likewise happen the 100th time a lady has engaged in sexual relations, brought about by things like little tears on the vaginal wall, feminine spotting, and a couple of different things like polyps in the vagina.

No matter what the subtleties of your sexual life systems and the bare essential insights concerning your hymen, a sexual accomplice ought to never cause you to feel terrible for any piece of your sexual history. Whether that implies they anticipate that you should be a virgin and you're not, or on the other hand assuming that you've never had intercourse and

 they have. It's savvy to examine history with another accomplice if you have a background marked by STIs, especially herpes, HPV, or another STI that isn't reparable.

Eventually, Jessica told the person she was dating about her own set of experiences since she would have rather not lain. Furthermore, assuming he'd responded ineffectively (he didn't), she would love to tell the truth. "You expect to accept me for who I am, past and all," she said.

CHAPTER 6

Does bleeding always occur?

Does a lady generally drain when she engages in sexual relations interestingly?

Actually no, not dependably. A few ladies will drain in the wake of engaging in sexual relations interestingly, while others will not. Both are typical.

A lady might drain when she has penetrative sex interestingly as a result of her hymen extending or tearing.

The hymen is a slim piece of skin that to some extent covers the entry to the vagina. For certain ladies, it might stretch or tear when they begin having intercourse.

Having an extended or torn hymen doesn't guarantee that a lady has lost her virginity.

The hymen can likewise stretch or tear effectively before a lady engages in sexual relations interestingly, through:

exercises, for example, horse riding and different games
utilizing tampons
masturbation
A lady may not have a clue about whether her hymen has extended or torn, because it doesn't necessarily cause torment or recognizable dying.

If you're worried about draining after sex, get counsel from a GP or your closest sexual well-being facility.

CHAPTER 7

How to make love to a virgin lady

Most ladies have had sufficient experience to know how to delight a man in the room, you should rest assured that there are a few young ladies who might be virgins when you initially bring them to bed.

However, most Indian men like to have intercourse with a virgin. There are additionally various men who hate the thought because of the tension of having intercourse with somebody with no experience.

So on the off chance that you end up dating a virgin, there are a couple of significant things that you ought to continuously remember when you take her to bed. However you have had intercourse with various ladies previously, and you want to figure out that this one being a virgin will realize hardly anything about what is generally anticipated of her in bed. Since she will be restless and apprehensive, you must be even more cautious to guarantee that she will partake in her most memorable time with you.

Kiss her

Whether you are doing it with a virgin or somebody with a record that would humiliate Pam Anderson, you ought to take as much time as necessary to have intercourse with her with your lips. Utilize your lips with energy, and kiss her parts that different folks will more often than not overlook. Kiss her lips, her hips, her shoulders, her hands, and cuddle her ears - parts which aren't required sexual.

Give your young lady a hand
OK, this one might gaze directly out of a B-grade south Indian film, yet getting going with an erotic full-body rub is an incredible approach to warming her up. So utilize a few pleasant fragrant oils like lavender or Yang to knead her body. On the off chance that you are more capable, you would know the different erogenous zones of a lady's body. Begin with the scruff of her neck and gradually work your direction down to her back, tenderly massage her bosoms and play with her areolas, delicately flick at them and control them to an erection.

Inspire her to lie on her stomach and back and rub her inward thighs. Affectionately stroke her bum and move your hands near her valley of joy. She may be excessively bashful to tell you, however, her definitive joy point would be kicking the bucket for your consideration.

Delicately, stroke her external lips or the labia. Whatever, misgivings or fears she might have had about sex will all vanish once your finger begins making wizardry in her lower areas.

Never scrutinize her
Keep in mind, that she has never felt a man's body, which implies that when she attempts to investigate your body you may not be guaranteed to appreciate it. So let her hold your penis and stroke it, let her lick and snack you and stimulate your body. You may not find her awkward considerations very stimulating yet don't cause her to feel like a beginner in bed.

If she accomplishes something right let her in on the amount you are getting a charge out of it. Guide her fingers to your pleasure focuses and tell her what you would like a young lady to do in bed. Being the more experienced accomplice you

 ought to resemble her caring tutor and show her the complexities of pleasuring a man.

Make her touch herself
While she might have stroked off previously, by inspiring her to contact herself you would have the option to cause her to feel the unexplored world. Tell her how severely you need to see her jerk off. The thought is open to her to possess sexuality.

Now is the right time to infiltrate
At the point when you believe that she is at long last fit to be infiltrated, enter her as tenderly as could be expected. Likewise, ensure that she is creating sufficient oil to work with the demonstration. Keep your strokes slow and shallow and abstain from pushing excessively profound during your initial not many strokes.

Assuming you can cause her to feel good and protected, any agony that she might insight initially will before long vanish and be supplanted by groans of bliss.

The initial time can be harrowing for most men. Simply recollect how apprehensive you were at the point at which you engaged in sexual relations interestingly. So when you take your virginal sweetheart to bed for the first time makes the experience as pleasurable for her as could be expected.

Remaining a virgin in a sex-fixated society can be a difficult errand. You'll observe that setting solid and sound individual limits is vital to keeping up with independence over your own body, and, further, to set the terms of what you endlessly are not happy with doing with an accomplice.

Section 1
Instructions to Characterize Your Limits
The picture named Biogenetic Individual Thinking
1
Think about your reasons. Understanding the reason why this choice is vital to you is a major piece of keeping up with it. Find an opportunity to inspect your thinking. Try not to be a virgin as a result of your parent(s), your strict chiefs, your accomplice.— be a virgin if it looks like what is reasonable for you.
Take a stab at posting your considerations in a diary, so you can take a gander at them at whatever point you feel like it.
Likely explanations behind declining incorporation...
Your strict, otherworldly, or individual convictions incorporate pausing or restraint.

You don't feel prepared or intrigued.
You're agamic, and you feel that sex sounds exhausting or gross.

You maintain that your most memorable time should accompany somebody extraordinarily.

You need admittance to contraception, boundaries, or sexual medical care.

You are underage or feel that you are excessively youthful. You have fears about your security: possibly you are frightened of pregnancy, STIs, and so on or your family is severe and your close-to-home well-being or well-being would be compromised on the off chance that they got you.

2
Consider your period.

For how long would you like to be chaste? A great many people don't carry on with their whole lives as virgins, and laying out clear and sensible objectives for yourself is great. Contemplate how long you need to remain a virgin, and realize that you can constantly change the choice on the off chance that it no longer works for you.

Choosing to be chaste for quite a long time is an excess of tension for certain individuals. Have a go at making a period restricted agreement with yourself (for example "I will be chaste this month"), and afterwards audit and conceivably recharge it toward the finish of every month.

Certain individuals like to hold on until marriage. This is alright. Simply recollect not to hurry into a marriage given your chemicals; marriage is a significant choice and you maintain that it should accompany the ideal individual!

3
Free yourself of any misinterpretations.

 Sex isn't malevolent, and forbearance won't make you "unadulterated" or ethically predominant. Sex can be delightful between consenting, genuinely pre-arranged grown-ups. It doesn't genuinely change your body, or change the way that you're a decent individual. Try not to allow your chastity to be driven by dread, yet rather by a solid and informed decision to stay away from sex.

The vast majority wind up having intercourse sooner or later in their lives. If eventually, you conclude that you're prepared, you shouldn't need to feel remorseful about it.

4
Characterize your terms.
 "Virginity" and "sex" are terms that different individuals characterize unexpectedly.
Before you can declare your limits, you want to know how you characterize these terms for yourself.
How would you characterize "sex"? What sort of close contact would you say you are alright with, and what is excessively far for you? How would you characterize "virginity"? Is it a profound, mental, or actual state or some mix thereof?
You'll have to have these boundaries set up for yourself so you'll understand what's acceptable for yourself and have the option to convey it plainly to other people.
Assuming that you know your limits, are positive about communicating them, and anticipate that they should be regarded, you'll be more engaged to go to bat for yourself and do what you feel is correct.

5
Characterize your energy decision.
 Rather than zeroing in on the disadvantages of sex, contemplate the beneficial things you will do.
If you won't have a sexual accomplice now, what else might you at any point invest your energy in?

To be a virgin until a specific period, work on that objective. For instance, if you needed to hold on until you felt more sure and decisive, then, at that point, attempt self-assuredness preparing and constructing your certainty.

6
Characterize your limits.
 You get to decide the particulars of your physical, close-to-home, and mental limits. No other person has an option to encroach on or slight your limits.
Decide your close-to-home limits. What sort of close-to-home contribution would you say you are agreeable and awkward with? What sorts of ways of behaving make you genuinely awkward? Be clear with yourself that others' sentiments are not a higher priority than your own.
Think about your psychological limits. How much would you say you are happy with letting others' thoughts and sentiments impact your own? When do you feel somebody isn't regarding your considerations or thoughts? How much do you feel open to making sense of or safeguarding your convictions to someone else?
Ponder your actual limits. How and where and when are you open to being contacted? What sort of actual contact crosses your limits? Lay out the details of your limits, both for you and other people.
There are agendas online to assist you with sorting out what you endlessly are not happy with.

7
Be OK with — and glad for — yourself and your own body.
We're much of the time encompassed by obstinate messages about how we ought to or shouldn't look, feel, and act. What's

more, those messages can cause challenges for us to feel legitimized and enabled in our own choices. However, assuming you're sure about yourself and your choices, you'll be enabled to anticipate that others should regard you and your decisions in your particular manner.

Try not to forfeit your solace or your limits on account of strain from another person. If somebody doesn't regard your limits,

 move away from them and quit investing energy alone with them. Define the boundary between what's satisfactory and what isn't, and request that they regard that.

8

Track down sound sources for repressed energy. Except if you are agamic, you might feel occurrences of sexual longing. Deal with your necessities and delivery your energy in manners that you feel alright with.

Work out: go for a stroll, play sports, or go around with some relatives.

A few virgins feel OK with stroking off.

Wash up, or utilize a hot or cold pack.

Track down things to zero in on past sex, whether it's a speciality, composing, companions, family, chipping in, or homework.

.

Section 2
Instructions to Convey Your Limits to an Accomplice

1

Be forthright with anybody you date. As far as some might be concerned, a sexless relationship is a huge issue, and it is just a tad unreasonable for both of you to put off letting them know your sex position. Tell them before things get excessively intense so that nobody's heart gets split assuming you are separate.

However, it might very well be enticing to put off telling an individual you like that you intend to keep up with your virginity but don't. They'll find out in the end. It's smarter to ensure you're in total agreement about your needs in a relationship before you get excessively connected.

On the off chance that the individual isn't in total agreement and can't be in that frame of mind without sex, that is OK — that is their decision to make. Be that as it may, don't feel compelled by their choices; commonly regard each other's choices. If you're not in total agreement, heading out in a different direction with no worries is OK.

2

Get some margin to discuss limits with your accomplice. Let them know what you are and aren't happy with, and let them let you know what their limits are. Assuming you need it, you might carve out an opportunity to clear up for them why keeping your virginity (for the present or perpetually) means quite a bit to you. They might be confused and have inquiries for you; you can carve out an opportunity to make sense of them on the off chance that you feel happy with doing such.

Assuming your accomplice attempts to arrange your limits with you, clarify that these are significant limits. Your accomplice needs to regard them.
To remain a virgin, simply say as much. An expression like "I'm not happy discussing that" works.

3
Be clear about assent in your relationship (for kissing and contacting). Assent is significant, and you want to know how to give it, pull out it, and assess whether you have it. It's essential to speak the truth about what you like and could do without. In a utilitarian relationship, you and your accomplice should convey obviously and pay attention to what the other individual says.

Say "no" or say you need to dial back when you begin feeling awkward. A straightforward expression such as "I could do without that," "I don't feel prepared for that," or "Not presently" makes it clear to your accomplice.

Be clear about saying "OK." Your accomplice ought to constantly understand what page you're on while you're doing things together. Verbally say OK, grin, visually connect, and play a functioning job.

Assuming you're questionable, simply say as much. An essential "I don't know" works, or you can be coquettish and

say "I don't have the foggiest idea. Might you at any point persuade me?"
Pose inquiries to your accomplice: "Do you like this?" "Consider the possibility that I...?" "Need to make out."

4

Practice your entitlement to say no. If anytime you feel awkward or questionable, say you need to stop or dial back. A decent accomplice takes a "no" truly and will promptly regard your sentiments.
You are permitted to express no whenever: including when you said OK five minutes prior, when you were alright with accomplishing something last week, or when every other person is good with getting it done. You can express no whenever and any spot.

Utilize the messed-up record method to battle pressure: continue offering something like "No" or "I would rather not."
If you are bashful, work on saying no. Take a stab at recording the expressions in this article and work on saying them. Saying no is a significant fundamental ability.

5

Remain solid assuming somebody pressures you. A deferential accomplice won't attempt to change your limits, yet not all individuals are conscious. You reserve the privilege to set the terms for your own body; on the off chance that the other individual doesn't regard those terms, they don't regard you. A straightforward "no" ought to be sufficient. Yet, on the off chance that it isn't, be ready for a portion of the pushback you might get. Certain individuals are not adequately experienced to hear things they could do without.

Keep your reaction brief, legit and aware (at first), and be ready to rehash it if important. You can utilize the messed-up record strategy, and that implies rehashing the same thing notwithstanding pressure (for example "No" or "I would rather not").

For instance, assuming somebody says, "On the off chance that you don't allow me to do this, it implies you don't cherish me." Answer by saying, "I love you and I don't believe you should contact me at present/in like that."
According to assuming somebody, "However you let me do this previously." Answer with "I reserve the privilege to alter my perspective.

According to assuming somebody, "You're simply a wet blanket (or cold or curbed or whatever)," answer with "I'm OK with myself and my body and I'm requesting that you regard that." On the off chance that somebody doesn't regard your limits or causes you to feel uncomfortable, this is an issue. It could be an ideal opportunity to address whether you need to be seeing someone that.

6
Leave assuming things go bad.
On the off chance that somebody will not regard your limits, either close to home, mental, or physical, leave. Figure out how to leave serenely and unhesitatingly. Mainly, you move away from that individual, at the same time, on the off chance that you can, attempt to pass on the circumstance with quiet and certainty to pass on the message that they can't control you.
If you're at a party or other get-together, leave them and track down a companion to converse with all things being equal. On the off chance that you're separated from everyone else or almost alone with the individual, leave and head off to

someplace where others are near or where you can find support assuming that you want it (stroll towards a crisis call box, towards a taxi, and so on.).
As you leave, envision folding up their words and discarding them.
After disposing of their words, say and embrace something sure about yourself.

7

Make them leave.
 If you're in a circumstance where somebody won't try to understand and drop the subject, there are a couple of reactions you use to emphatically urge them to get lost. Assuming you're at a party, a bar, or another circumstance where somebody isn't tolerating that no, you're not intrigued, you reserve each option to look at them dead without flinching and say, "I said no. If it's not an extremely big problem, leave." If you have any desire to get some entertainment out of the circumstance and you don't think this individual is genuinely a danger (if you truly do feel undermined, move away from them and find help right away), you can express something like, "I get ridiculously, super connected to somebody assuming I engage in sexual relations with them," or "I'm not prepared to educate you regarding my herpes status."

Section 3
The most effective method to Oppose Companion Strain

1
Comprehend the sorts of companion pressure.
It's probably nothing unexpected to you that teenagers face peer pressure, including strain to engage in sexual relations. To all the more likely to oppose peer pressure, it assists with having the option to remember it or what it is. At the point when you perceive that somebody's utilizing one of these strategies, you can all the more likely set yourself up to stand up. The significant sorts of friend pressure are:

Clear companion pressure: This is the plainest type of tension and it normally includes immediate, unsubtle explanations from others like, "I can't completely accept that you're not having intercourse. Every other person is!"

Devious companion pressure: This is the sort of strain that is a smidgen more inconspicuous and is generally used to cause you to feel like there's something peculiar or amiss with you for not adjusting. It could sound something like, "It doesn't matter, you're a virgin, so you don't have the foggiest idea" or alluding to you as "the virgin" "the stick in the mud," and so on.

Controlling companion pressure: This sort of strain is an obvious endeavour to constrain you to do something by taking steps to bar you or end the fellowship on the off chance that you don't do what the other individual needs. It could sound something like, "We can't be companions if you're not kidding" or "I don't spend time with virgins."

2
Have one or two serious doubts.
Individuals around you might boast, yet it's probably they're misrepresenting while perhaps not out and out lying about what they get up to.
However, they might appear to be persuading, training yourself to have doubts about what others guarantee they've done. You don't need to call them on it essentially, yet you ought to document what they say under "most likely false."

3
Know the goodness of the expression "that is false." It may very well be hard to keep up with your feeling of satisfaction and self-assurance notwithstanding pessimistic outside messages, whether they come from media, mainstream society, companions, families, or authority figures.
Assuming somebody attempts to test your limits with negative remarks or proclamations that you realize aren't correct, persevere. Rehash the expression "That is false!" either to yourself or the following person until the memo sinks in.

4

Characterize the ramifications of engaging in sexual relations for yourself. Frequently a huge piece of friend pressure has to do with causing it to appear like having intercourse implies explicit things, as if you have intercourse you become a grown-up or are in some way or another freer of your folks.

Try not to acknowledge others' evaluation of what your sexual status implies about you. This might be especially significant if you're in secondary school, where friend tension about sex can be difficult to disregard. Try not to allow individuals to attempt to let you know things like, "on the off chance that you haven't

engaged in sexual relations this is because you're not joking" or "on the stand that you're not bluffing," and so on. Deciding not to engage in sexual relations implies none of those things. It implies you're making the right decision for you actually and inwardly.

5
Encircle yourself with positive individuals. An incredible method for diminishing pessimistic companion pressure is to avoid individuals who cause it.

Assuming you have companions who pester, ridicule you, or in any case pressure you about sex, ask them serenely and without hesitation to stop. On the off chance that they don't, quit spending time with them so much.

Find and spend time with companions who are tolerating your decision and regard your entitlement to choose for yourself.

6
Leave.
Similarly as with managing an accomplice who isn't regarding your limits, you can and ought to likewise leave a companion who isn't regarding those limits.

Leave smoothly and with certainty. Mainly, you move away from that individual, yet, on the off chance that you can, attempt to leave what is happening with quiet and certainty. That way you're imparting to them that they can't control you.

As you leave, envision folding up their words and discarding them.

In the wake of disposing of their words, say and embrace something certain about yourself.

7

Regard everybody's all in all correct to pick and don't disgrace individuals for pursuing decisions not quite the same as yours. Try not to sex disgrace or strain individuals to be like you. Sexual action is a strong private decision, and similarly, as you regard other people who partake in a functioning sexual coexistence, they ought to regard you for keeping away from sex.

Master question and answer session

Pose an Inquiry

What is your inquiry?

Tips

If somebody won't take "no" for a response, it very well may be an indication that they don't genuinely regard you or your independence. In the direct outcome imaginable, it might be an indication of an oppressive individual, and you ought to consider moving toward somebody you trust for help.

Recall that you and you alone get to decide your limits. On the off chance that somebody can't or won't regard those limits, you reserve the privilege to ask, or on the other hand, if important, demand, that they avoid you.

Assault and sex are various things. Assault is a demonstration of savagery and control, while sex is a demonstration of want. You can be an assault survivor and a virgin.

.

Specialist, I want your assistance to explain an issue, which has been giving me a restless night. I'm a virgin of 29 years and single. Kindly let me know whether being a virgin at 29 years is dangerous. On the off chance that indeed, what are the dangers?

I helped this data through a companion that it is exceptionally unsafe for a lady to stay a virgin for this long, and from that point forward I have been extremely stressed. Saying thanks to you for your expected to comprehend and early reaction.

From K.

On an overall outline, my response will be both a direct and a roundabout.

For one's purposes, restoratively talking, no extraordinary gamble joined to is being a virgin at age 29 years similarly as not be guaranteed to put you at a superior position for each future conceptive movement.

Optimistically, notwithstanding, is the way that it sets you in a place of virtue according to the difficulty of reaching the numerous physically communicable diseases. Remarkable among these are the significant ones like HIV/Helps, Syphilis, Hepatitis B, Chlamydia and Gonococcus diseases.

Other physically communicable contaminations that you are safeguarded from while you keep up with the virgin status

incorporate herpes simplex infection (type 2), and initial moles.

Besides these, it tends to be induced that you are better shielded from the chance of creating disease of the cervix (the cervix is the entry waterway into the belly or uterus). This is so because exploration discoveries are highlighting the way that early first sexual (particularly before the age of 16 in women) and ensuing repetitive sex put such women at a higher gamble for the improvement of cervical disease further down the road. The disease of the cervix gets developed further down the road and thus it is an ordinary person in old ladies in their mid-fifties ahead.

Likewise fascinating to note is the significant data that HIV/Helps is a significant gamble factor for the improvement of disease of the cervix in ladies of more youthful age bunch. Subsequently, since sex is a significant road that HIV is reached from, going without sex through virginity maintenance is likewise twofold insurance from HIV/Helps and by deduction right off the bat set malignant growth of the cervix.

Social wise, particularly in societies nearby, it truly deserves note that it is the longing of men to meet their significant other on their most memorable night together after their marriage.

Albeit, the orientation disadvantage here is somewhat on the lady, where the constancy of the hymen (the Virginia layer covering of the vagina) is a certain indication of virginity upkeep, in any case, no such identical sign exists in the male.

Subsequently, assuming that the reason for staying a virgin is to keep up with the indication of virtue for your man in future, nature doesn't appear to be sufficiently caring to give the same

 sign in the man that will console the lady worry that her man has likewise been as unadulterated as she has been.

Then again, nonetheless, I ought to express that there are a few laid out discoveries that for the most part highlight the way that late first pregnancy in quite a while put them at a higher gamble for a few pathologic circumstances, no matter what the way that the lady has kept up with her virgin status or not.

Unmistakable among such pathologic circumstances is the higher probability of creating Fibroids in the uterus of ladies who had their most memorable pregnancy late in their regenerative life. As such, the old clinical proverb which says that belly that couldn't convey infants will ultimately convey a fibroid is a more clear clarification of this turn of events.

Likewise, reviewing careful exploration of discoveries on the gamble factors for bosom disease additionally highlights the way that early and repetitive pregnancies in ladies are defensive against the improvement of bosom malignant growth in future. Here as well, the gamble isn't virginity status related.

In this way, getting disciplined a lot later in the contraceptive existence of a lady may not be defensive against the improvement of bosom malignant growth in future.

Along these lines, more seasoned pregnant ladies (especially, those over 35 years) are more in danger of having children with inherent irregularities than ladies who get pregnant at a more youthful age; the same for different difficulties in pregnancy.

From the previously mentioned, my sincere exhortation according medico-social perspective is that similarly as it is

 alluring to keep up with the virgin status in light of the prior referenced coincidental benefits, it's anything but a mutually beneficial arrangement, particularly as for deferring early pregnancy.

1. Virginity implies various things to various individuals
Nobody is meaning to virginity. For some's purposes, being a virgin method you haven't had any sort of penetrative sex — whether that is vaginal, butt-centric, or even oral. Others might characterize virginity as never captivating in vaginal entrance with a penis, regardless of having had different kinds of sex, including oral excitement and butt-centric entrance.

Anyway, you characterize it, the main thing to recollect is that you choose when you're prepared to engage in sexual relations and that you're OK with that decision. Furthermore, when that opportunity arrives, do whatever it takes not to consider it "losing" or "giving" something away. You're acquiring a different encounter.

2. Regardless of whether your idea of virginity includes entrance, there's something other than P in V
Many individuals trust the best way to "lose" your virginity is through the vaginal entrance with a penis, however, that is not the situation.

Certain individuals may never again call themselves a virgin in the wake of participating in the butt-centric entrance or entrance with a finger or sex toy. Others might revaluate their virginity status after getting or giving oral excitement. With regards to virginity and sex, there's far beyond only P in V.

3. On the off chance that you have a hymen, it won't "pop" during vaginal infiltration
Gracious, the hymen — the stuff of legend. You've likely heard the fantasy that if you have a hymen, it will break during the vaginal entrance. Yet, that is all that is: a fantasy.

The typical hymen isn't a piece of level tissue that covers the vaginal opening, similar to the legend claims. All things being equal, it's normally a free — and not by any stretch of the imagination unblemished — piece of tissue that stays nearby the vagina.

Contingent upon its size, a hymen can be torn during penetrative sex, exercise, or other actual work. Be that as it may, it won't "pop," since it just can't.

4. Your hymen doesn't have anything to do with the situation with your virginity
Your hymen — like your finger or your ear — is only a body part. It doesn't decide if you're a virgin or anything else than your toes do. Furthermore, not every person is brought into the world with a hymen, and if they are, it could be a tiny piece of

tissue. You — and you alone — choose the situation with your virginity.

5. Your body won't change
Your body doesn't change after you engage in sexual relations interestingly — or second, or third, or 50th.

Nonetheless, you will encounter specific physiological responses connected with sexual excitement. This might include:

- enlarged vulva
- erect penis
- quick relaxing
- perspiring
- flushed skin

These excitement-related reactions are short-term. Your body isn't changing — it's simply answering the improvement.

6. There isn't a post-sex "look"
After you're done engaging in sexual relations, your body will gradually get back to its normal state. Be that as it may, this cool down period just endures a couple of moments.

All in all, it's now assuming that you choose to tell them.

7. It presumably won't resemble the intimate moments you see on television (or in pornography)
Everybody unexpectedly encounters sex. Be that as it may, you shouldn't anticipate that your most memorable time should resemble what you find in the motion pictures.

Simulated intercourses in movies and TV don't occur in one take — entertainers frequently need to reposition themselves, and chiefs might reshoot specific parts so the scene looks great on camera.

This implies that what you see in the cinema regularly is certainly not a reasonable image of what sex resembles for a great many people.

8. Your most memorable time might be awkward, yet it shouldn't do any harm
It's considered common to feel awkward whenever you first engage in sexual relations. Contact might occur with entrance, and that could cause uneasiness. However, your most memorable time shouldn't do any harm.

Assuming that having intercourse harms, however, that could be a result of an absence of grease, or conceivably an ailment, like endometriosis. You ought to see a specialist on the off chance that you experience torment each time you have intercourse. They can survey your side effects and assist with treating any basic circumstances.

9. This is where oil (and perhaps some foreplay!) comes in
On the off chance that you have a vagina, you might deliver oil — or become "wet" — normally. Yet, some of the time, there may not be sufficient vaginal grease to lessen grating during infiltration.

Utilizing lube can assist with making vaginal intercourse more agreeable by limiting disturbance. Assuming you're participating in the butt-centric entrance, lube is a flat-out must; the rear end doesn't deliver grease of its own, and the entrance without oil can bring about tears.

10. Your sheets most likely won't be horrendous

There might be some light draining whenever you first have intercourse, however, don't expect a scene from "The Sparkling."

If you have a vagina, you might encounter minor draining assuming your hymen extends during the entrance. Furthermore, on the off chance that butt-centric channel tissue tears during butt-centric infiltration, gentle rectal draining may happen. In any case, this ordinarily doesn't create sufficient blood to leave a wreck on the sheets.

11. Physically communicated diseases (STIs) can be spread through any sort of sex

Vaginal infiltration isn't the main way that STIs are spread. STIs can likewise spread through the butt-centric entrance and oral excitement, whether or not you're giving or getting. That is the reason it's essential to utilize condoms and different types of insurance each time, without fail.

12. If you're having P in V sex, pregnancy is conceivable at the initial time

Pregnancy is conceivable whenever there is a vaginal entrance with a penis, regardless of whether it's your most memorable time. It can work out on the off chance that an individual with a penis discharges inside a vagina or outside, yet close, the vaginal opening. Utilizing a condom is your most effective way to forestall pregnancy.

13. On the off chance that you have a vagina, you may not climax the initial time
Climaxes aren't generally an assurance, and there's an opportunity you may not peak whenever you first have intercourse. That could occur for various reasons, including solace levels and ailments. Research recommends that 11 to 41 per cent of individuals with a vagina experience issues arriving at the climax with an accomplice.

14. If you have a penis, you may climax quicker than you anticipate
It is entirely expected for an individual with a penis to peak quicker than they expected — or needed — during sex. Concentrates on demonstrating the way that untimely discharge can influence upwards of 1 out of 3 individuals.

If you climax rapidly each time you have intercourse, think about conversing with a specialist. They might have the option to endorse prescriptions or suggest different treatments.

Alternately, it's likewise conceivable that you may not encounter a climax whenever you first have intercourse, regardless of whether you discharge.

15. Or on the other hand you might observe that your penis is uncooperative
You might observe that you can't get or keep an erection firm enough for entrance. Even though you might feel humiliated or upset, know that infrequent erectile brokenness (ED) is entirely expected.

ED can occur for various reasons, like pressure and tension. Furthermore, because this is whenever you're first having intercourse, you might feel a ton of uneasiness.

On the off chance that ED continues, you might find it supportive to converse with a specialist about your side effects.

16. The more agreeable you are, the more probable you are to climax
You're bound to climax when you're OK with your body, your accomplice, and the experience overall. At the point when you're agreeable, you become more responsive to sexual excitement. Thus, you're bound to feel pleasurable sensations all through your body. What's more, throughout sex, those sentiments could develop into a climax.

17. However, climaxes aren't generally the point,
Try not to fail to understand the situation — climaxes are perfect! They cause floods of delight all through your body that cause you to feel far better. In any case, having a climax isn't generally the place of sex. What makes the biggest difference is that you and your accomplice are both agreeable and similarly to the experience you're having.

18. If you need something, say as much
Try not to overlook your longings. Assuming you have specific needs and needs, try to tell your accomplice — as well as the other way around. It's vital to be transparent about what you

might want to happen whenever you first have intercourse so the experience is all that it tends to be.

19. You don't need to do anything you're not happy with
No means no. Full stop. On the off chance that there's something you're not happy with doing, you don't need to get it done. Your accomplice doesn't reserve the option to pressure or power you into having intercourse — as well as the other way around. Furthermore, this doesn't just apply to your most memorable time — this goes for each time you have intercourse.

Assuming your accomplice says no, this isn't a greeting for you to continue to inquire. Requesting that somebody accomplish something again and again with the expectation that they'll give in is a type of compulsion.
20. You can alter your perspective anytime
You don't need to keep having intercourse on the off chance that you're as of now not happy or intrigued. You reserve the privilege to alter your perspective anytime. Once more, your accomplice doesn't reserve the option to compel or force you into proceeding to engage in sexual relations on the off chance that you would rather not.

21. as it were "ideal opportunity" is the point at which it feels appropriate for you
You might feel strain to have intercourse sooner than you're truly prepared to. It's memorable critical that you're the one in particular who can choose when you need to engage in sexual relations interestingly. Assuming the timing feels off, that is fine. Hold on until it feels ideal for you.

22. Whether "every other individual is getting it accomplished" is distant from being valid

In all honesty, every other person isn't getting it done. The pace of individuals engaging in sexual relations is going down. As per one 2016 review, 15 per cent of Recent college grads haven't engaged in sexual relations since they were 18 years of age.

Furthermore, information from the Communities for Infectious prevention and Anticipation shows that more young people in the US are holding on to engage in sexual relations interestingly. The typical age today is currently around 17 years of age, up from 16 years of age in 2000.

23. Sex isn't inseparable from closeness or love
Sex, such as running, is actual work — and that's it. It isn't the same thing as closeness, love, sentiment, or a profound bond. How you view sex, however, is a touch more perplexing. Certain individuals may just have intercourse with accomplices whom they love, while others might have intercourse without any hidden obligations.

At the end of the day, you ought to ensure you're alright with the reality that you're having intercourse, and that the other individual may not share any upright or profound worth you might put on the experience.

24. Your spirit isn't in question, nor will it be connected to that individual until the end of time
Certain individuals might have areas of strength for having convictions around sex. Others may not. One way or another, you won't imperfection your spirit from engaging in sexual relations, nor will you be for all time bound to your accomplice. Eventually, sex is only that — sex. It's a typical, sound movement that doesn't characterize or decide your moral or otherworldly establishment.

25. Assuming you have intercourse with somebody you consistently interface with, the dynamic might change
You and your accomplice both might be left posing new inquiries, for example, "Do we need to do this each time we see one another?"; "Is sex continuously going to be that way?"; and "What's the significance here for our relationship?" A percentage of the reactions might be convoluted, yet as you communicate about these topics, make a position to stay transparent about your emotions.

26. Your most memorable time doesn't establish a vibe for the sex you could proceed to have
The incredible thing about sex is that it's an alternate encounter like clockwork. Your most memorable time engaging in sexual relations may not satisfy your hopes, but rather that doesn't mean the second, third, or fourth time will as well. The kind of sex you could conceivably proceed to have will rely upon the accomplice, level of involvement, eagerness to attempt new things, and thus considerably more.

27. On the off chance that your most memorable experience isn't what you needed, once more, you can constantly attempt
Your most memorable time having intercourse doesn't need to be a limited time offer movement except if you pick so. If the experience isn't what you needed or expected, once more, you can constantly attempt — and once more, and once more, and once more. All things considered, as the expression goes: Careful discipline brings about promising results.